Gestational Diabetes

Step by Step Understanding, Managing, and Preventing Diabetes in South Asian-Indian Women During Pregnancy

Table of Contents

Introduction

I dedicate this book to all mothers-to-be by sharing information I gathered on the topic of Gestational Diabetes for last decade and a half. I first came across the term 16 years back when I was diagnosed with the health condition.

I was detected with gestational diabetes in the second trimester of my pregnancy with my first child. The doctor mentioned that it was a condition that mostly affects South Asian women owing to their lifestyle, diet, and genetic make-up. Although I tried my hardest to remain calm, my anxiety got the better of me, and I ended up frantically looking for information on the Internet.

I quickly realized that there was a dearth of relevant and applicable information about Gestational Diabetes in South Asian- Indian women, and it was difficult for a patient to get answers to her questions. That's when I decided to pen down my experience to help all those that are in need of some guidance during their pregnancy. If you are an Indian woman like me, then it is important for you to understand the risks of developing the illness and how you can successfully combat it, like I did.

I am a complete vegetarian and based in the US. Having to deal with a tough job that required me to travel four days a week made my pregnancy a little harder than most other women. If you, too, are in a similar situation in your life, then this book will be your gestational diabetes guide. It is aimed at helping women understand the importance of maintaining a proper diet and also taking care of their bodies during pregnancy.

I have conducted extensive research on the topic and present to you all of the valuable information in a condensed format. You will find this book particularly informative and useful, considering that there are very few books and mini books available on the topic. However, please note that this book is solely based on personal experience and in no way should be considered a medical journal of any sort. Let us begin!

Chapter 1: What is Diabetes Mellitus?

First and foremost, I wish to thank you for choosing this book and hope it serves the intended purpose of educating you on the topic of gestational diabetes. In this first chapter, we will look at the meaning of diabetes mellitus or simply, diabetes.

Diabetes mellitus is a metabolic disease that causes blood to contain excess amounts of sugar. This sugar is nothing but a breakdown of the food that is consumed on a day-to-day basis. The body needs a certain degree of energy to operate normally and acquires it by breaking down the glucose that is present in foods.

Once the food is broken down, and the glucose is separated, it passes into your bloodstream and remains there until the body uses it up. But your body's cells cannot directly process the glucose from your blood and require help from a hormone known as "Insulin." Insulin assists the body in absorbing the glucose by opening up the cells.

Once the cells open up, insulin then guides the glucose into the cells to help them function optimally. However, a person suffering from diabetes mellitus will suffer from an insulin imbalance, causing the blood sugar levels to spike. The imbalance can either be one where the body does not produce enough insulin to be absorbed by the cells, or the insulin itself is not working towards dissipating the glucose in the body.

Either way, the result will be that of high levels of glucose present in the bloodstream, as the cells in your body do not acquire any of it. Patients with elevated levels of blood glucose end up having it pass through their urine, which gives the illness its name "diabetes mellitus" meaning "sweet urine."

There are two types of diabetes, and they are as follows.

Type-1 diabetes

Type-1 diabetes occurs in young adults and children and is also sometimes known as juvenile diabetes. Around 5% of the population in the world suffers from this type of illness.

Type-1 diabetes occurs as an autoimmune disease where the cells that produce insulin are permanently disabled by the person's immune system. These cells are present in the pancreas, and the patient's body will be unable to produce enough insulin to dissipate the glucose.

It is imperative for people suffering from this type of diabetes to take proper medication to lead a healthy life. According to According to Wild S, Roglic G, Green A, Sicree R, King H, 2004, South Asians are at least risk to develop this form of diabetes with just 1-2% of the populace being at risk.

Type-2 diabetes

The other form of diabetes is known as Type-2 diabetes. This is more common amongst South Asians and one of the most widely spread illnesses in the world. Type-2 diabetes is a condition where the bloodstream accumulates a lot of glucose over the course of several years. If not checked on time, Type-2 diabetes can damage the body from the inside and cause the person to lead a painful life. Therefore, early diagnosis is the key to preventing diabetes-related complications.

As mentioned earlier, our bodies require energy to perform day-to-day activities. This energy is a result of the glucose that is broken down inside through the digestive system. This glucose is then transported to the different cells of the body by a hormone known as insulin. Insulin is chiefly responsible for opening up the cells and depositing the glucose inside the cells. However, when these cells become less responsive to insulin, the pancreas start producing large doses of the hormone, all in a bid to help the released glucose to be absorbed by the cells

This causes the insulin in the body to work abnormally, causing the entire system to backfire. Your body ends up having smaller doses of insulin circulating in the blood, unable to work towards transporting the glucose to the cells. This, in turn, causes your bloodstream to remain high on glucose, at all times.

In the earlier days, Type-2 diabetes was mostly seen as an illness that affected adults and was known as the adult-onset diabetes. However, times have changed, and the early onset of obesity in children has made the disease one of the most widespread illnesses in the world. Common symptoms of diabetes include fatigue, increased urination, insatiable thirst, blurred vision and extremely dry eyes. Many reasons can contribute towards the onset of Type-2 diabetes including obesity, stress, hereditary factor, smoking, drinking, consuming oily, unhealthy foods, etc.

Why South Asians are at most risk of developing Type-2 diabetes?

As per research studies, South Asians are at most risk of developing diabetes owing to the diet and genetic make-up. Let us look at some of the main reasons for the development of diabetes in South Asians.

Diet and obesity

Most South Indian foods are rich in fat and sugar. These can lead to obesity, which causes the onset of Type-2 diabetes. People, especially women, are at greater risk if the obesity occurs around the lower part of the abdomen.

Genes

Genes are also chiefly responsible for the onset of diabetes. As per a study conducted in 2011, 6 different types of genes are responsible for the start of diabetes.

Fat burning

It is believed that most South Asians end up burning fat that lies in their muscles and not their cells. This can further increase the risk of developing Type-2 diabetes.

Indians and diabetes

Indians are at the highest risk of developing diabetes and India is known as the diabetic capital of the world. It is estimated that there are more diabetics in India than the entire collection of diabetics around the world.

This is mostly owing to the diet and lifestyle choices that Indians are exposed to. The traditional Indian diet is supposed to have been well balanced with equal proportions of carbohydrates, proteins, and fats. However, due to excessive urbanization, the Indian diet has gone for a toss and people end up consuming unhealthy foodstuffs.

Most Indian diets consist of foods laden with fats and sweets are eaten during every meal. This heightens the risk of Type-2 diabetes and affects all age groups.

Sedentary lifestyles and the lack of physical activities also contribute towards the development of Type-2 diabetes.

It is, therefore, important for Indians to exercise caution and try to remain as prepared to stave off diabetes as possible. It is of particular importance for pregnant women to be proactive to prevent gestational diabetes.

Chapter 2: What is Gestational Diabetes?

In the previous section, we understood the basics of diabetes and also saw why Indians are at the highest risk of developing the illness.

In this chapter, we will discuss the meaning of gestation and gestational diabetes.

What is gestation?

Gestation refers to the conception of a child. It occurs when the man's sperm successfully fertilizes the woman's ovum. Gestation period refers to the period that the pregnancy lasts. Humans have a gestational period of 40 weeks or 9 months. The gestational period is divided into 3 trimesters incorporating 3 months each.

The first trimester starts from the first day of the last period and goes into the 13th week of pregnancy. Most women are unaware that they are pregnant until they miss a period. This is the time when women must take good care of their bodies as the fetus is at most risk. Most miscarriages occur during this stage of pregnancy. Many women feel extremely uneasy during this period and develop morning sickness, nausea, and fatigue.

The next 3 months are known as the second trimester of pregnancy. This is the time when most women recover from the above symptoms and regain vital vigor. The baby starts to develop, and the woman can feel the baby's kicks. It is also possible to determine the sex of the baby at this stage of pregnancy. The last semester stretches over the last 3 months of pregnancy. This is when the fetus completely develops, and the baby takes up all the available space in the womb. At the end of 9 months, a woman enters labor and delivers a baby after about 24 hours.

Gestational diabetes

Gestational diabetes is a condition that occurs during pregnancy. Women that have never had diabetes before but high blood sugar it during pregnancy are said to suffer from gestational diabetes. It is believed that 10-25% women are in danger of developing this type of diabetes. There is no conclusive proof to determine what exactly contributes towards the development of gestational diabetes, but here is a plausible explanation.

During pregnancy, the placenta provides nutrition to the baby and causes him or her to develop properly. But the placenta can block the release and absorption of insulin, which can contribute towards the onset of insulin resistance.

This resistance causes the woman's body to have increased levels of blood sugar during the pregnancy.

Here are some terms that you must acquaint yourself with, to better understand the concept of gestational diabetes.

- Glycemic index

Glycemic index refers to a particular food's capacity to increase the level of sugar in the blood. Each food has a different glycemic index with sugar having the highest capacity.

- Glycemic load

Glycemic load refers to the amount of carb that a particular food contains. Starchy foods have the highest glycemic load.

- Insulin index

Insulin index relates to a combination of the above two and the capacity of food to raise blood sugar after two hours of consumption.

Although Gestational Diabetes starts during pregnancy, lasts the course and subsides after birth, the woman remains at risk of developing full-fledged Type-2 diabetes if she does not take good care of herself.

Gestational diabetes in South Asian women

As per recent studies, there has been a spike in the number of gestational diabetes patients around the world (10-15%), with South Asian women being at the highest risk (15-25%). But research has also found that women in some areas of Asia have a greater risk of developing GD as compared to women based in certain other parts of Asia, such as India (20-25%).

For instance, as per a study done in New York, the frequency of South-Asian women (Sri Lankan, Indian, Fijian Indian, Pakistani,) suffering from GDM is usually higher than that of South-East Asian women (Cambodian, Laotian, Filipino, Vietnamese, Thai, Malaysian) and East-Asian women (Chinese, Taiwanese South Korean, and Japanese).

Women from South Asia who have migrated to foreign countries also run an equal risk of developing the condition. This is owing to the prevalence of genes that can target the onset of the condition.

Chapter 3: Symptoms and Risks of Gestational Diabetes

Gestational diabetes is a condition that affects 15% of pregnant women. South Asians, Indians especially, run the highest risk of developing this form of diabetes (15-25%). So, only women who are pregnant will run the risk of developing this type of diabetes and not regular women. Most pregnant women with gestational diabetes will not be able to tell that they are suffering from it.

The initial symptoms include thirst, dry eyes, and fatigue. But since these are symptoms of normal pregnancy, many women are unable to say whether they are suffering from gestational diabetes. However, if you suspect that you are having unusual bouts of these symptoms, then it is best to have your blood tested to check for gestational diabetes.

Effects on baby

Although most mothers with gestational diabetes give birth to healthy babies, there is always a certain element of risk to be wary of. Here is how GD can affect your baby.

- Macrosomia. Macrosomia is a condition where the baby's body is unusually large. This can be a problem during delivery. The woman might have to undergo a cesarean to deliver the baby.

- Hypoglycemia. Hypoglycemia refers to low sugar levels in the baby's bloodstream. This might necessitate a compulsory breastfeed right after the birth of the baby.

- Jaundice. Jaundice is when the baby's skin turns yellow and can cause discomfort. The illnesses can be limited with treatment.

- Respiratory distress syndrome. Respiratory distress syndrome is where the baby finds it difficult to breathe.

- Another effect of GD on the baby might include low levels of calcium and magnesium in the body of the baby.

Apart from these, your baby might be a little uncomfortable post birth, and the doctor might have to check for any of these symptoms. But most of them can be tackled with ease.

It is believed that those women who develop GD in their 30's are more prone to developing Type-2 diabetes post-partum.

Some important points to note:

If you have been diagnosed with gestational diabetes, then it is important for you to exercise a little precaution. Here are some things to know about it in advance.

- If you have taken insulin injections during your pregnancy, then you will have to take it during your labor and pregnancy as well. But if you haven't then you can avoid it or ask your doctor about the same. It is usually administered through a plastic tube that runs through your arms.

- Women with gestational diabetes have a higher risk of developing preeclampsia, which tends to induce high blood pressure during the third trimester. If that happens, then it is extremely important for women to be as cautious as possible to avoid complications in childbirth. It can also lead to early birth.

- Some women with gestational diabetes might also have to deliver their baby through C-section or cesarean. This calls for your stomach and womb to be cut open to pull out the baby.

Post-partum

Many women with gestational diabetes wonder if they will have diabetes after giving birth to their baby and the answer in most cases is no. Your body will be able to produce and use insulin more efficiently after you give birth. This will help your body bounce back and combat the condition effectively. However, this might not always be the case as you might develop Type-2 diabetes if the insulin resistance continues inside your body. The experts state that women who were detected with Gestational Diabetes have a 35 to 60% risk of developing Type 2 diabetes within five to ten years.

You need to speak with your doctor about the same to know if you will remain at risk of developing the condition and what is best for your body.

But remember, it always bests to stay proactive, and we will look at how you can remain so in the next chapter.

Chapter 4: Being Proactive

Remember that it is important to be as proactive as possible in order to both avoid complications during birth and developing diabetes later. Here are some things that you can do to stave off complications and the risk of developing Type-2 diabetes.

When it comes to managing gestational diabetes, you have to adopt a two-tiered approach. The first step is to know the amount of blood that exists in your bloodstream and the second step is to manage it effectively. Once you do both, you will have the chance to control your risk of developing diabetes post birth.

Knowing your sugar levels

When it comes to understanding your sugar levels, you have to ensure that you check it yourself from time to time. To do so, you can buy yourself a self-testing kit. You can buy it from a drugstore or also order it online. But ensure that you buy a good brand that gives you near accurate results.

Checking at regular intervals

Remember that it is extremely important for you to check your sugar levels from time to time to ensure that it is well within the normal range. Your body will have varying levels of sugar in the blood stream depending on what you eat when you eat and also the physical activities that you take up. In general, your body's sugar levels will spike up as soon as you consume food and should ideally come down around 2 hours after you have your last meal.

Keeping track of your blood sugar levels will help you know what foods can be eaten and when. For example, checking every day after breakfast will tell you whether you can have ½ a bagel more or it will negatively impact your body. This helps in taking care of your cravings and prepares you to better combat the onset of Type-2 diabetes. It also helps you know exactly when your sugar levels are high and what you can do to bring it down effectively.

Self-testing

Here are easy steps that you can follow to test your blood sugar level using a self-testing kit.

1. The first step is to wash your hands with warm water and soap as it helps soften your skin.

2. Next, use the small needle (lancet) provided with the kit to poke the top of your right index finger. This finger is generally preferred by a majority of people but you can also pick another finger that you deem fit.

3. You can then gently press the area around the prick to build up on the released droplet of blood.

4. Next, you must carefully place the drop of blood on the glucose strip that is provided with the testing kit.

5. Insert it into the testing machine and wait for 5 to 10 seconds for the meter to read your sugar level.

6. Record the reading or make a note of it and maintain a regular record of the same.

Remember that it is important to check your sugar levels from time to time to ensure that it remains within the specified range. Here are the times when you have to check your glucose level.

- Fasting glucose level—this is done as the first thing in the morning before eating or drinking anything.

- Postprandial--1 or 2 hours after breakfast, make sure you don't do it earlier or later

- 1 or 2 hours after lunch

- 1 or 2 hours after dinner

You have to record the readings after each session to know exactly how your body is coping with the raised sugar levels.

The chart here is to help you to check if your sugar levels are within the ideal range.

Fasting glucose level - No higher than 95
One hour after eating - No higher than 140
Two hours after eating - No higher than 120

Don't worry if your levels are higher than these, you can speak with your doctor and seek advice to combat it.

Remember that stressing over it only causes the sugar level to increase and it is best for you to continue to be as calm as possible in such situations.

Chapter 5: Controlling Gestational Diabetes with Diet and Physical Activity

When it comes to controlling the sugar levels in your blood, you have to work on both nutrition and physical activity.

Diet

As you know, the food we eat is composed of several types of nutrients, all of which contribute towards helping the body function optimally. But one nutrient, in particular, can help control gestational diabetes to a vast extent.

Carbohydrates are what give the body energy to perform day-to-day activities. However, consuming too much can mean supplying the body with too much glucose, which is not entirely used up by the body. It can cause a spike in the blood sugar levels and heighten the risk of developing Type-2 diabetes. It is important for you to work closely with your doctor, nutritionist or health care provider to create a nutritional plan that helps in regulating the amount of carbs that you intake.

It is important for you to calculate the carbs for every meal that you eat to make sure that your body is availing the ideal amount. It is essential for you to ensure that it lies within the specified range and is not too much or too little.

You can also choose the exchange system of consuming food. It refers to exchanging one nutrient rich food for another like tofu for chicken, without affecting the carbohydrate level. But ensure that you pick foods that are allowed within your food plan and consult your nutritionist before making the exchange.

It is also very important for you to increase the level of fiber in your diet. Fiber helps in burning away a lot of the glucose, thereby reducing its presence in the blood stream.

It is also important for you to snack from time to time. Research has shown that doing so helps in controlling blood sugar levels to a large extent. But make sure you snack on healthy foods such as fresh vegetables and fruits.

It is essential to avoid the consumption of junk and processed foods as they are mostly laden with sugar. They will spike up your blood sugar level and put you at risk of developing Type-2 diabetes. You can always prepare healthier versions of the foods at home and not have to worry about compromising on your cravings.

The combination of right nutrition and the correct amount of physical activity helps you keep gestational diabetes under control. In this chapter, I hope to give you an insight of how to manage these two critical aspects so that you can overcome challenges associated with gestational diabetes thereby helping you deliver a healthy, bonny baby while you maintain your good health too.

For a better understanding of the nutritive contents in your food, allow me to take you through various nutrients that you get from the food you consume. Moreover, while none of the nutrients can be left out of your daily diet, it is imperative that you make wise choices so that you and your baby have access to a balanced diet and remain healthy.

Understanding Carbohydrates

You must be careful to make sensible food choices by knowing and understanding how much of carbohydrate is given by the food you eat. Split your carbohydrate intakes into bite-sized options, each of which will give you approximately 15 grams of carbohydrates. For example, one carbohydrate choice will equal to 15 grams of carbohydrates, two carbohydrate choices will be 30 grams of carbohydrates and so on and so forth.

The following list gives you an idea of the relationship between carbohydrate choices and carbohydrate grams:

Carbohydrate choice	Carbohydrate (grams)
½	6-10
1	11-20
1 ½	21-25
2	26-35
2 ½	36-40
3	41-50
3 ½	51-55
4	56-65

The following list is an example of foods that contain 15 grams of carbohydrates:

- Frozen or canned fruit – ½ cup
- Fish - 4 oz
- Fresh fruit - 4 oz
- Bread – 1 slice
- Tortilla – one 6-inch
- Oatmeal – ½ cup
- Crackers – 4-6

- English muffin – ½
- Starchy vegetable of black beans – ½ cup
- Baked Potato – 3 oz
- Fat-free yogurt (plain or with sugar substitutes) – 2/3 cup
- Cookies – 2 small
- Cake or brownie (without frosting) – 2-inch square
- Sherbet or ice cream – ½ cup
- Honey, sugar, jelly, jam – 1 tbsp.
- Light syrup – 2 tbsp.
- Chicken nuggets – 6
- Casserole – ½ cup
- Soup – 1 cup
- Medium French fries – ¼ of a serving

For example, the following 3 items would give you about 90 grams of carbohydrates.

- Chicken nuggets and a cup of soup – 6 (for lunch)
- Baked Potato – 6 oz (for breakfast)
- Fresh fruit – 4 oz with a tbsp. of honey drizzled over (a snack)

Using the above data, you can arrive at your own diet to include the daily required carbohydrate intake.

Understanding Fats

Fats, like carbohydrates, are energy providing nutrients for our body. However, unlike carbohydrates, their calorific value is twice that of carbohydrates so the intake of fats requires to be closely monitored. You cannot leave out fats from you daily diet, as the body needs them for purposes other than providing energy.

Fats are primarily are of two types: saturated fats and unsaturated fats.

- Saturated fats: At room temperature, saturated fats are usually solid. They are found in abundance in animal-based foods such as eggs, hamburgers, butter, and bacon. Your saturated fat intake should not be more than 10% of your total daily calorie requirements.

- Unsaturated fats: At room temperature, unsaturated fats are usually liquid. These fats are typically found in many vegetable oils such as those extracted from olive, canola, sunflower seeds, almonds, peanuts, and avocados. Unsaturated fats are also sourced from cold-water fish like albacore tuna and salmon. You must keep intake of unsaturated fats at a moderate level.

Because you need to keep your fat intake under check, the following tips will help you to achieve this end:

- Ensure you remove the fat and skin from chicken before you eat

- Use grilling, roasting, baking, boiling, or baking methodologies to cook instead of frying in fat or oil

- Remove all visible fat from meats before eating

- Use as little oil for cooking as you can and make sure you choose vegetable oils instead of butter and oil extracted from animal products

- As nonfat and low-fat cheeses contain lesser amount of saturated fats, it makes sense to choose these over the usual cheeses

- Similarly, use nonfat and low-fat milk and yogurt

- Try and avoid butter and margarine or at least keep the usage to a minimum

- It is better to use herbs and spices in your pasta, meats, and vegetables instead of gravies and sauces

- Before buying processed foods, check for fat content and avoid those with excessive fat and sugar content

- Use low-fat checkers and pretzels instead of cookies and chips.

Understanding Protein

Essential nutrients for your body, proteins are vital for the growth and repair of cells and in the gestation period, the function of growth and repair of cells take high priority within your body. Remember the following the main aspects of proteins:

- Proteins do not affect the level of glucose in your blood -a great piece of news for all you pregnant women struggling to manage gestational diabetes. Ensure you include 3 servings of protein every day

- With very little amounts of saturated fats, consuming nuts and seeds daily is an excellent way to get proteins into your system

- A fully cooked egg is a great source of protein and is very easy to include in multiple meal plans

- While fish is an excellent source of protein and is also low in saturated fats, there are precautions to be taken as types of fish carry the risk of enhanced mercury levels.

- Nonfat and low-fat cheeses are great providers of protein to your body.

Understanding Fiber in your Diet

Fibers in your diet have the power to lower blood glucose levels because they slow down digestion as well as nutrient absorption. The following foods are excellent sources of fibers:

- All whole-grain foods are rich in fibers. When you buy processed foods such as bread, pasta, tortillas, and crackers, remember the ingredients must say, "Made with 100% whole grains." Choose only these foods to be included in your diet.

- Fresh fruits are also rich in fiber content, and it is more prudent to choose fresh fruit over juices. Moreover, many citrus fruits such as tangerines, oranges, and grapefruit are excellent sources of Vitamins C and A, both of which are vital nutrients during pregnancy.

- Deeply colored veggies such as orange, deep yellow, dark green, and red vegetables are great foods to be included in your diet during gestation as they contain many essential nutrients. Ensure you include broccoli, spinach, carrots, romaine, and peppers in your daily diet.

- Legumes such as beans and peas are high sources of fiber content

Apart from the macronutrients mentioned above, other essential micronutrients need to be part of your daily diet during gestation. And these include:

- **Vitamins-** A prenatal multivitamin taken daily supplies the daily vitamin needs for both you and your growing baby. Ensure you choose one which contains iron, calcium, and folic acid as these extras is required by you and your child

- **Fluids-** It is critical to stay hydrated and for this, you need to drink about 8-10 glasses of fluids a day. Keep your fruit juice intake to less than 50% of your total fluid intake; this helps in keeping gestational diabetes under check. Completely avoid aerated sodas and artificially flavored drinks.

- **Calcium-** Remember that the baby growing in your womb needs to get calcium for the growth of her or his bones from you. So, the inclusion of extra calcium is imperative in your pregnancy diet. Make sure you include milk and dairy products, as they are excellent sources of calcium. However, considering the need to keep fat intake under control, ensure you choose nonfat and/or low-fat milk. If you are lactose intolerant, include other non-dairy calcium-rich foods such as collard greens, rhubarb, spinach, etc. in your diet. Calcium supplements can also be taken.

Besides the care you need to take regarding foods and nutrients that you consume during your pregnancy, there are additional points to consider preventing avoidable untoward health-related incidents from happening either to you or your beloved baby. Here are a few more precautions you need to take about food:

- **Sugars** – Perhaps, the primary aspect related to gestational diabetes, it is imperative that you control your sugar intake and ensure that you do not cross the limit set by your doctor. Choose low-calorie sweeteners like sucralose, aspartame, acesulfame-potassium and other such sweeteners that are considered safe for use by pregnant women. Pregnant women are advised to avoid Saccharin-based sweeteners as these cross the placenta.

- **Caffeine** – It is better to keep caffeine intake to less than 6 ounces per week during the entire period of pregnancy

- **Alcohol-** Abstaining from consuming alcohol during the entire period of gestation is highly recommended. Prenatal alcohol exposure can lead to development delays and birth defects.

By this point, you have a better understanding of how much and what kind of nutrients are right for you and your baby and what foods to definitely avoid or at least minimize the intake. So let us move on to how you can optimize physical activity to keep gestational diabetes under check and within manageable proportions such as the health of you and your baby are not negatively affected.

Physical Activity

One good way of curbing the weight gain and diminishing the effect of GD is to perform physical activities. Physical activity not only helps in controlling the sugar levels abut also makes you happy. It can aid in staving off stress, which is a precursor to Type-2 diabetes.

Here are some dos and don'ts of physical activity that you can ponder over.

The Importance of Physical Activity

- You have to take up a moderate physical activity that helps you feel calm and relaxed. But consult your healthcare provider before taking up any new activity.

- One of the best physical activities to take up when pregnant is swimming. Swimming helps in massaging your organs and also aids in controlling weight gain. You don't have to stand up for too long and can avail an easy exercise.

- Moderate physical activity is required on a regular basis. An ideal schedule would be 30 minutes per day for 5 days a week. This kind of daily activity has the potential to reduce insulin resistance thereby helping in the prevention of undue weight gain. When you are exercising, make sure your heart rate does not exceed 140 beats per minute.

- If you can get this activity done within an hour or two after a meal, then your postprandial blood glucose levels will see a significant reduction. For best results, keep the physical activity after your largest meal of the day.

- Ensure that you do not get carried away by the various TV shows, friends, and relatives, etc. giving you tips for better weight management and other such non-professional advice. Stick to an exercising plan that is customized and fixed for you (to meet your individual needs and assessment) by a professional service provider.

- One way to check if you are exercising the right amount is to speak and see if you are able to do so fluently.

- It is important to wear the right type of clothing to remain comfortable. Pick light clothing that will let you breathe easily and prevent you from sweating too much or getting too hot.

- If you are feeling hot or the weather outside is hot, avoid exercising as this could lead to dehydration. Moreover, during your physical activity, remember to stay well hydrated.

- It is best for you to carry a water bottle with you when you go to your physical activity. Remaining as replenished as possible helps in availing better results. You can also consume fruit infused water to replenish your body.

- Try to eat the highest amount of carbs just before your workout session so that your body has a chance to burn it away quickly.

- Avoid exercising without eating a proper meal or after you have fasted. It is entirely wrong to deny nutrition both for yourself and your baby. Ensure you keep your schedule of physical activity as advised by fitness professionals and doctors.

- Remember moderation is crucial. Be sure not to over exert and that you can breathe easily and normally without much effort. Do not go to such an extent that exercising makes you feel fatigued. You have to be aware of your surroundings and feel alert during the entire workout session.

- Avoid doing those exercises that need you to lie on your back when you are in your second and third trimester. Lying flat on your back can be uncomfortable for your baby

- Avoid activities that create any kind of imbalance and have the potential to knock you over. These risky ventures can cause physical harm to both yourself and to your baby

- If you have any of the following medical conditions, then avoid physical activities entirely: intrauterine growth restriction, preeclampsia, vaginal bleeding, abruption or placenta previa

So, to summarize, a combination of moderate and regular physical activity and a balanced intake of nutrients is essential to keep gestational diabetes at bay and to have a healthy and joyful pregnancy. It is only when you are fit physically and mentally that your baby will grow healthily so that at the end of the complete term, you will rejoice that bundle of joy that will be in your hands.

Chapter 6: Maintain a Healthy Weight Gain

Remember that it is natural for you to gain weight when you are pregnant, but it is essential to know whether you are gaining the right amounts. If you suspect that you are getting overweight quickly then it might be owing to gestational diabetes.

While it is very natural to gain weight during pregnancy, it is also important to track and check the weight gain. If the weight gain is more than expected or is not within allowed limits, then it could be because of gestational diabetes. It is important that you maintain a healthy weight gain during pregnancy.

Weight gain during pregnancy is monitored in two different ways; one is overall gain and the other is a weekly rate of increase. It is not uncommon for some health care professionals to rely only on the overall gain. However, there are many professionals to keep a check on both the regular and the overall.

Let us first understand the concept of overall weight gain. A health overall weight gain is dependent on what your body weight was before the pregnancy. Use the following table to find out which category you belonged to regarding height and weight before pregnancy.

The last row of the table gives you an indication of what a healthy weight gain ought to be. These figures are merely a benchmark, and there could be changes depending on various other factors including your age, your genetic makeup, your body mass index, your individual physicality, and more.

Height (without shoes)	Pre-pregnancy weight (in pounds with light indoor clothing)			
	A	B	C	D
4 feet 9 inches	92 or less	93-113	114-134	135 or more
4 feet 10 inches	94 or less	95-117	118-138	139 or more
4 feet 11 inches	97 or less	98-120	121-142	143 or more
5 feet	100 or less	101-123	124-146	147 or more
5 feet 1 inch	103 or less	104-127	128-150	151 or more
5 feet 2 inches	106 or less	107-131	132-155	156 or more
5 feet 3 inches	109 or less	110-134	135-159	160 or more
5 feet 4 inches	113 or less	114-140	141-165	166 or more
5 feet 5 inches	117 or less	118-144	145-170	171 or more
5 feet 6 inches	121 or less	122-149	150-176	177 or more
5 feet 7 inches	124 or less	125-153	154-181	182 or more
5 feet 8 inches	128 or less	129-157	158-186	187 or more
5 feet 9 inches	131 or less	132-162	163-191	192 or more
5 feet 10 inches	135 or less	136-166	167-196	197 or more
5 feet 11 inches	139 or less	140-171	172-202	203 or more
6 feet	142 or less	143-175	176-207	208 or more
Your overall weight gain goal is:	35-40	30-35	22-27	15-20

Why is it important to keep track of weight gain during pregnancy?

While for people who do not have gestational diabetes, it can easily be stated that weight gain is because they eat more food than they need, with gestational diabetics, this need not necessarily be the case. When you have gestational diabetes, too much of weight gain or weight loss could be a symptom of something going wrong with your body. And because the insulin functioning is already compromised, ignoring this symptom could lead to avoidable negative health conditions both for you and your baby.

When and How to manage and ensure a healthy weight gain?

It is best for you to start managing your gestational weight gain as soon as you realize you are pregnant. And you have to keep track of your weight throughout your pregnancy till you deliver your baby. Keeping track and letting your doctor know about any weight-related abnormalities (no matter how seemingly small) gives you the huge advantage of detecting, treating, and managing any health-related issues thus keeping you and your baby safe.

While regularly recording your weight, it is important to note the following points so that your readings are consistent and abnormalities are clearly visible:

- Weigh yourself without footwear
- Weight yourself with similar light indoor clothing every time
- Make sure you stick to the same day of the week and same time of the day for checking your weight

Moreover, your weight will be checked and recorded during your pre-natal checkups with your gynecologist.

The ways and means to manage your weight gain have already been spoken of in the previous chapters. Just to reiterate, two aspects that need to be considered simultaneously to achieve healthy weight gain during pregnancy include regular moderate physical activity and following a healthy, balanced, low-fat diet.

How to track if you are on the right path?

Perhaps, the best way to see if you are in the right direction when it comes to healthy weight gain is to check if your weekly weight gains are in order and as per health requirements. Some health care providers treat this record as equally important as the record of overall weight gain. This is because the weekly rate history gives you an idea as to whether your diet and physical activity schedule are helping to control and manage gestational diabetes.

If there are significant or regular abnormalities in your weekly rate, then your diet and physical activity can be altered suitably. If your weight gain per week is too low, then your diet could be adjusted to increase calorie intake, and if your weight gain per week is too high, then you could potentially be heading towards preeclampsia, a medical condition that can be dangerous for both you and your baby.

Here is table giving you some indicative figures of what your weekly weight gain should ideally be:

In the first trimester or the first 3 months of your pregnancy	3-6 pounds for each week of the *entire three months*.
During the 2nd and 3rd trimesters or the last 6 months of your pregnancy	About ½-1 pound each week.
If the weight gains in the initial trimester is excess	Ensure your weight gain in the last 6 months is restricted to about 3/4 pound per week (or 3 lbs every month). This will keep gestational diabetes under control.

Remember gaining 2 pounds or more a week is high and is not healthy at all, and weight gains are not uniform throughout the pregnancy. Some weeks, you may be put on more pounds than what is indicated in the above table and some weeks, you may not have gained any weight at all. Your doctor is your best adviser regarding telling you whether your weight gain is within limits, or too high, or too low, and make appropriate changes in your physical activity schedule and diet.

However, it is vital for you to remember that weight losses can be very dangerous. Please report any weight loss to your health care provider and/or doctor immediately so that he or she can take corrective measures to prevent further complications.

Ways and means to keep and maintain a healthy. weekly weight gain

Here are a few tips that will help you achieve a healthy weekly weight gain plan:

- Ensure you stick to a moderate and regular physical activity plan as advised by your health care provider

- When you are buying packaged foods, ensure you read the nutrition facts on the label and make healthy food choices

- Avoid or minimize intake of fried or fast foods

- Include healthy dishes such as salads with low-fat dressings, grilled or broiled chicken, and less of butter and margarine in your diet.

- Make sure you replace sauces with herbs and spices in your pasta, rice, and other foods.

- Make sure you eat smaller quantities of low-calorie food frequently rather than large amounts of high-calorie food and less often. For example, eat 5-6 meals and snacks (keep track of overall daily calorie intake) instead of just breakfast, lunch, and dinner. This ensures that you do not get starved.

- Ensure you do NOT avoid any meals especially breakfast and lunch. Avoiding or skipping meals makes you hungrier and hence you end up overeating instead of eating right.

Keeping and maintaining records

It is vital for you to note down all the critical elements that can affect gestational diabetes. These records help you and your care provider arrive at the correct balance of diet and physical activity that will assist in controlling gestational diabetes. These elements include:

- What you eat at every meal – This record should meticulously include every bit that you consume. Do not leave anything out. In fact, make a note of what you see on your plate and then eat it. That way you will not forget to record what you consume throughout the day. Nitpicking as it may sound, these small details could be the difference between managing gestational diabetes and letting it go out of control.

- Your physical activity details – Ensure you make a note of what physical activity including the time and duration.

- Your glucose levels – Checking and keeping a record of this element is critical to see whether the plans of diet and physical as prescribed by your health care provider are working well or not. Adjustments can be made only when these recordings are correct and reflect the actual status. It is important to stick to the same time of the day to monitor and track the movement of glucose levels in your blood.

What if the diet plans and the physical activity schedule is not helping in the management of gestational diabetes?

If after diligently following the diet plans and fitness programs as prescribed by your doctor, you find that your blood glucose levels are not being controlled well, then it might make sense to include insulin treatment. However, this has to be done ONLY under the advice and prescription of your authorized health care provider. The following conditions usually call for the inclusion of insulin treatment to manage gestational diabetes:

- Very high levels of blood glucose

- Blood glucose levels are spiking too frequently

- Blood glucose levels are high, but there is no weight gain and/or it is not safe for you to do physical activity

While the above are some of the indications for insulin, there could be other factors too; however, to reiterate an earlier point, it is critical to take insulin only under the supervision of an authorized medical professional. Self-medication is a complete no-no!

It is equally important to know that taking insulin does not absolve you to having to maintain a healthy low-fat diet and an approved physical activity plan. Insulin is an added treatment and rarely excludes all other ongoing therapies like a balanced diet and moderate physical activities.

Low Sugar

Remember that low sugar is just as bad as high sugar and is something that you must be aware of. Low sugar can cause discomfort and can also cause you to faint. So it is essential to maintain the right sugar level at all times. Some of the causes of low sugar can include skipping meals, exercising too much, injecting too much insulin.

Here are some special instructions if you are advised insulin treatment and how to avoid low sugar:

- Strictly follow a regular eating pattern consisting of a balanced inclusion of all essential nutrients

- Be aware of the symptoms of low blood glucose levels, which if they go below 60 is called hypoglycemia and can be potentially very dangerous. Low blood glucose levels can be caused by excessive exercise, skipping snacks and/or meals, delaying meals, not eating as frequently as you should, or excessive insulin. Report these low-sugar levels immediately to your doctor and he or she will find alternative methods to bring back normalcy.

- The symptoms of low-sugar include feeling fatigued, feeling famished, trembling or shaking, clamminess or excessive sweating, feeling or nervousness and/or confusion, blurred vision, and feeling faint.

What are the chances that your diabetic condition will continue or recur after you have delivered your baby?

While gestational diabetes usually goes away once you deliver your baby, it is possible that you may develop diabetes later too. There are a few elements that increase the recurrence of type 2 diabetes within 5 years of having your child. The traits that can trigger a recurrence include:

- Gestational diabetes appeared before the 24th week of pregnancy
- Blood glucose levels are always towards the higher end of the allowed range
- Blood glucose levels were greater than average even after delivery
- Diabetes runs in your family
- Gestational diabetes appeared even other pregnancies too
- You belong to impaired glucose tolerance category and/or belong to a high-risk ethnic race such as African American, Hispanic, South or East Asian, Native American, and other such groups

If one or more of the above is true for you, then please consult your doctor, seek medical advice, and take early precautionary measures. It is quite likely that you can develop diabetes later on.

Future pregnancies

Plan your future pregnancies well. Test yourself for blood glucose levels and ensure they are well within the normal range at least 3 months before you conceive to prevent any issues later on. After you conceive, make sure your doctor is aware of your history of gestational diabetes so that he or she can factor it into future courses of action.

Conclusion

I thank you once again for choosing this book.

My primary intention for writing this book is to bring awareness to South Asian – Indian women on the importance of being prepared for gestational diabetes. Although it proved to be a blessing in disguise for my family and I, as the food habits I adopted during pregnancy helped put us on the right track, it is still quite important to treat it as a serious health threat.

While I was devastated when I first heard that I have gestational diabetes, in retrospect, I now appreciate that it was a blessing in disguise for my family and me. The healthy lifestyle habits including well-balanced meals and physical activity schedules were something that I continued even after my pregnancy and these practices have ensured that my blood glucose levels are well within the normal range.

Managing my weight, working out regularly, and making healthy food choices were amazing habits picked up during those difficult times and they have stood me in good stead. The painful yet highly revelatory journey of gestational diabetes proved to be an eye-opener for me and made me acutely aware of this epidemic that is threatening to take our world apart. These fears are especially true for Asians, as many studies have unequivocally revealed for reasons already shared in the early chapters of this book.

It is important, therefore, as responsible citizens of the world to set an example for the future generations and make sensible lifestyle choices that do not jeopardize our health. As we work toward setting correct standards, we will definitely see our young children follow these steps too and thus be assured of a long and healthy life on this beautiful planet.

Remember to remain proactive and give your body the chance to recuperate with ease.

Good luck!

CREATE YOUR CUSTOMIZED DIET PLAN TEMPLATE - 1500 CALORIES

- ✓ STARCH (Carbs) – 7   (One Serving- 80 Cals)
- ✓ VEGETABLES – 4   (One Serving – 30 Cals)
- ✓ FRUIT - 1   (One Serving – 60 Cals)
- ✓ MILK - 2   (One Serving – 90-100 Cals)
- ✓ PROTEIN - 8 OZ   (One Serving- 35-55 gms)
- ✓ FAT - 4   (One Serving – 5 gms)

Meal	Type of Food	Food Taken	Calorie	Total Calories/meal
Breakfast	1 Carb		80	140 cals
	1 Protein		55	
	1 Fat		5 gms	
	Free	2 tsp sugar free jam/jelly		
Snack	1 Protein		55	115 cals
	1 Fruit		60	
Lunch	2 Carbs		160	440 cals
	2 Proteins		110	
	2 Veggie		60	
	2 Fat		10	
	1 Milk		100	
Snack	1 Protein		55	135 cals
	1 Carb		80	
Dinner	2 Carbs		160	435 cals
	2 Protein		110	
	2 Veggie		60	
	1 Milk		100	
	1 Fat		5	
Snack	1 Carb		80	135 cals
	1 Protein		55	

Gestational Diabetes

TEMPLATE TO DAILY TRACK YOUR BLOOD GLUCOSE LEVELS

Month		Morning		Breakfast				Lunch				Dinner			
Day	*Date*	*Time*	*Glucose*	*Time*	*Before*	*Time*	*After*	*Time*	*Before*	*Time*	*After*	*Time*	*Before*	*Time*	*After*

ABOUT THE AUTHOR

Ragini is a mother, an accomplished higher education executive, small business owner, and a social entrepreneur. She is the founder of a nonprofit organization called *Global Each One Teach One* dedicated to providing educational opportunities for children across nations.

Ragini has written this book on Gestational Diabetes with the intention to empower and create awareness among South-Asian Indian communities about the significant health impact it has on mothers, their children, their families, and their communities. Gestational Diabetes is affecting Indian (by 20-25%) and South Asian communities in the world at a rate significantly higher compared with women of various other ethnicities. Experts also state that these women who are afflicted with Gestational Diabetes have a 35 to 60% risk of developing Type 2 diabetes within five to ten years.

Please support Ragini in her Gestational Diabetes awareness initiative by buying this book for someone you know who will benefit from the information. All the proceeds from the sale of this book will be spent to create an awareness campaign for rural women in India in collaboration with a Senior Dietician specialized in Diabetes Management from John Hopkins Medical Center, USA, and a Senior OBGYN Doctor from Osmania Medical Hospital, India.

You can find us at

- www.fixgestationaldiabetes.com
- www.gestationaldiabetes.in
- https://www.facebook.com/Pushraj-Publications-226412667760819/